SHIATSU MASSAGE FOR HEALTH

Essential Manual To Relieve Pain, Reduce Stress, And Boost Wellness With Expert Techniques And Natural Healing Methods

Disclaimer:

The data in this book, "Acupuncture Therapy Simplified," is solely meant to be informative and instructional.

This book is not intended to replace expert medical advice, diagnosis, or care. No medical, health, or other professional services are offered by the author, publisher, or any affiliated parties

Individual outcomes may differ in the practice of these therapies, which entail a variety of approaches and methodologies.

A one-on-one session with a trained or certified healthcare professional is still preferable. It is best to consult a trained healthcare provider before making any decisions regarding your health.

The author of this book is not affiliated with any specific website, product, or organization related to any of these therapies.

All reasonable measures have been taken by the author and publisher to guarantee the authenticity and dependability of the material contained in this book.

Contents

"Shiatsu Massage for Health: A Guide to Japanese Bodywork" is a comprehensive exploration of the profound benefits and techniques of Shiatsu, an ancient Japanese therapeutic practice. This guide delves into the roots of Shiatsu, tracing its origins and elucidating its key concepts, while clearly distinguishing it from other therapeutic modalities. Readers will gain insights into how Shiatsu's unique approach to energy flow and meridian stimulation can be applied to enhance overall health and well-being.

This book provides an in-depth look at the meridians and acupressure points, fundamental components of Shiatsu. Understanding these concepts is crucial for effective application, as the guide covers essential acupressure points and techniques to stimulate them. It demonstrates how manipulating these points can influence energy flow, offering practical techniques to integrate into daily routines.

In addition to traditional Shiatsu techniques, the guide offers valuable information on self-Shiatsu practices. Readers will find detailed instructions for self-treatment, including preparation, key areas for focus, and step-by-step routines. This section empowers individuals to harness the benefits of Shiatsu independently, using tools and tips to enhance their practice.

The book also addresses Shiatsu's effectiveness in treating common ailments, from headaches and back pain to digestive issues and anxiety. It explores how Shiatsu can be tailored to meet personal health needs and improve mental well-being, providing techniques to alleviate stress, enhance sleep quality, and boost mental clarity.

For those engaged in physical activity, the guide highlights Shiatsu's role in sports and exercise. It outlines benefits for athletes, including muscle recovery and injury prevention, and offers practical advice for pre- and post-workout sessions.

Partner Shiatsu techniques are also covered, emphasizing preparation, communication, and creating a conducive environment for shared practice. This section illustrates how Shiatsu can strengthen relationships while promoting relaxation and mutual benefit.

Lastly, the book addresses common concerns and FAQs, clarifying misconceptions, session expectations, and safety measures. It guides on finding qualified practitioners and maintaining an effective Shiatsu practice, ensuring readers have a thorough understanding and practical resources at their disposal.

Introduction to Shiatsu

Shiatsu is a traditional Japanese form of bodywork that has its roots deeply embedded in ancient Chinese medicine and philosophy. It involves the use of finger pressure on various points of the body to enhance physical and mental well-being. Shiatsu is based on the principle of balancing the body's energy flow, known as "Qi" or "Chi." By applying pressure to specific points, practitioners aim to improve the flow of energy, alleviate pain, and promote overall health.

The practice of Shiatsu integrates principles from both Eastern and Western medical traditions. It combines the techniques of acupressure with the concepts of energy meridians, which are channels through which energy flows in the body. Shiatsu sessions typically involve the use of gentle but firm pressure, stretching, and manipulation of the body's soft tissues.

Understanding Shiatsu and its Origins

Shiatsu, which translates to "finger pressure" in Japanese, is a modern development of ancient techniques. It emerged in Japan during the early 20th century, influenced by traditional Chinese medicine, Western anatomical knowledge, and Japanese therapeutic practices. The practice was formalized by Shizuto Masunaga and Tokujiro Namikoshi, who adapted and systematized techniques to fit contemporary needs.

The origins of Shiatsu can be traced back to the practices of acupressure and acupuncture used in Chinese medicine over 2,000 years ago. Chinese medicine emphasizes the flow of vital energy, or Qi, through the body's meridians. Shiatsu adopted these principles and integrated them with Japanese massage techniques, creating a unique therapeutic approach that addresses both physical and emotional health.

Key Concepts of Shiatsu Massage

Shiatsu massage is grounded in several key concepts that guide its practice. Understanding these concepts can help you appreciate how Shiatsu works and its potential benefits.

Meridians: These are pathways through which Qi flows in the body. Shiatsu focuses on stimulating specific points along these meridians to enhance energy flow and restore balance.

Pressure Points: Similar to acupuncture points, these are specific locations on the body where Shiatsu practitioners apply pressure. Each point corresponds to different organs or systems within the body.

Energy Flow (Qi): The central concept in Shiatsu is the flow of Qi, which is believed to be crucial for maintaining health. Blockages or imbalances in Qi flow can lead to physical or emotional issues.

Balance and Harmony: Shiatsu aims to balance the body's energy and harmonize its systems. By restoring balance, Shiatsu helps improve overall health and well-being.

Holistic Approach: Shiatsu treats the whole person rather than just specific symptoms. It considers physical, emotional, and spiritual aspects to promote comprehensive healing.

Benefits and Applications

Shiatsu massage offers a range of benefits that can enhance both physical and mental health. Here are some of the key benefits and applications of Shiatsu:

Pain Relief: Shiatsu is effective in alleviating chronic pain, including back pain, neck pain, and headaches. By targeting pressure points and improving energy flow, Shiatsu helps reduce muscle tension and discomfort.

Stress Reduction: The calming effects of Shiatsu help to lower stress levels and promote relaxation. The practice encourages deep breathing and a sense of calm, which can be beneficial for managing stress and anxiety.

Improved Circulation: Shiatsu enhances blood flow and lymphatic drainage, which can improve overall circulation and support the body's natural healing processes.

Enhanced Flexibility: The stretching and manipulation techniques used in Shiatsu can increase joint flexibility and improve range of motion, which is particularly useful for athletes or individuals with stiffness.

Boosted Immune System: Regular Shiatsu sessions can strengthen the immune system by promoting overall health and balancing the body's energy.

Emotional Balance: Shiatsu addresses emotional well-being by releasing tension and promoting a sense of inner balance, which can be particularly helpful for managing emotional stress and enhancing mood.

How Shiatsu Differs from Other Therapies

Shiatsu stands out from other therapeutic practices due to its unique approach and techniques. Here's how Shiatsu differs from other therapies:

Pressure vs. Manipulation: Unlike many forms of massage that focus on kneading and manipulating muscles, Shiatsu primarily uses finger pressure and stretches to influence energy flow and balance.

Holistic Focus: While many therapies target specific symptoms or areas of discomfort, Shiatsu adopts a holistic approach that considers the entire body and its energy systems.

Energy Work: Shiatsu is deeply rooted in the concept of energy flow (Qi), which is not always a primary focus in other therapeutic practices. It emphasizes restoring balance and harmony in the body's energy.

Clothing and Touch: Shiatsu is typically performed through loose clothing, which differentiates it from therapies that involve direct skin contact. This approach can be more comfortable for some individuals and allows for a different type of therapeutic touch.

Integration with Eastern Medicine: Shiatsu incorporates principles from traditional Chinese medicine and Japanese practices, which sets it apart from Western therapies that may not emphasize energy flow or meridians.

Who Should Consider Shiatsu?

Shiatsu can be beneficial for a wide range of individuals, though it may not be suitable for everyone. Here are some groups who might benefit from Shiatsu:

Individuals with Chronic Pain: Those suffering from conditions like back pain, joint pain, or headaches may find relief through Shiatsu, which targets specific pressure points to alleviate discomfort.

People Undergoing Stress: Shiatsu is an excellent option for those experiencing high levels of stress or anxiety. The relaxation techniques used in Shiatsu can help manage and reduce stress.

Athletes and Active Individuals: Those who engage in regular physical activity may benefit from Shiatsu's ability to improve flexibility, reduce muscle tension, and enhance overall recovery.

Individuals Seeking Holistic Care: Shiatsu is suitable for those interested in a holistic approach to health that addresses both physical and emotional well-being.

Those with Emotional Imbalances: People dealing with emotional stress or imbalances may find that Shiatsu helps promote a sense of calm and emotional stability.

Individuals with certain medical conditions or those who are pregnant need to consult with a healthcare professional before undergoing Shiatsu to ensure it is appropriate for their specific needs.

CHAPTER ONE

THE MERIDIANS AND ACUPRESSURE POINTS

Overview Of Meridians In The Body

In Shiatsu massage, understanding the concept of meridians is crucial. Meridians are invisible pathways through which the body's vital energy, or "Qi," flows. These pathways connect different organs and tissues, creating a network that supports overall health and balance. Think of meridians as energy highways that transport vital energy throughout your body, ensuring that each part receives what it needs to function optimally.

There are twelve primary meridians, each associated with a specific organ system. These include the Lung, Large Intestine, Stomach, Spleen, Heart, Small Intestine, Bladder,

Kidney, Pericardium, Triple Burner (San Jiao), Gallbladder, and Liver meridians. Each meridian follows a particular route and influences the corresponding organ and its functions. For example, the Liver meridian travels from the big toe up the inner leg, through the abdomen, and ends at the chest, impacting the liver and its related functions.

Important Acupressure Points

Acupressure points are specific locations on the meridians that can be stimulated to influence the flow of Qi and promote healing. These points are like energy taps that, when activated, can help restore balance and alleviate discomfort. Some key acupressure points used in Shiatsu include:

L.I.4 (He Gu): Located on the back of the hand, between the thumb and index finger. This point is commonly used to relieve headaches, neck pain, and stress.

P6 (Nei Guan): Situated on the inner forearm, about two finger widths above the wrist crease. This point helps with nausea, anxiety, and digestive issues.

ST36 (Zu San Li): Found just below the kneecap, on the outer side of the shinbone. It is known to boost energy, improve digestion, and strengthen the immune system.

BL23 (Shen Shu): Located on the lower back, near the second lumbar vertebra. This point is associated with the kidneys and helps with lower back pain and fatigue.

How Energy Flow Works

Energy flow, or Qi, is central to Shiatsu massage. Qi is believed to flow through the meridians, nourishing the organs and tissues and maintaining harmony in the body. When Qi flows smoothly, you feel healthy and balanced. However, if there are blockages or imbalances in the flow, it can lead to discomfort or illness.

Shiatsu aims to restore the natural flow of Qi by using pressure and stretching techniques. By applying pressure to specific acupressure points, a Shiatsu practitioner can help release blockages and enhance the flow of Qi. This process can improve circulation, reduce muscle tension, and promote overall well-being. It's like clearing a traffic jam on an energy highway, allowing everything to move more freely and efficiently.

Techniques To Stimulate Acupressure Points

Stimulating acupressure points effectively requires a combination of techniques. Here are some commonly used methods:

Pressing: Apply firm, steady pressure with your fingers, thumbs, or palms to the acupressure point. This technique helps release tension and stimulate energy flow.

Rotating: Use circular motions to massage the acupressure point. This method can help increase blood flow and enhance the point's effectiveness.

Tapping: Lightly tap the point with your fingertips. This technique is useful for stimulating energy and awakening the body's natural healing abilities.

Stretching: Gently stretch the area around the acupressure point. This can help open up the energy pathways and improve flexibility.

Each technique can be adapted based on the specific needs of the individual and the condition being treated. A skilled Shiatsu practitioner will choose the appropriate technique and apply it with the right amount of pressure and duration to achieve the desired results.

Commonly Used Points In Shiatsu

In Shiatsu, certain acupressure points are frequently utilized due to their broad range of benefits. Some commonly used points include:

L.I.4 (He Gu): Besides its use for headaches and stress, it is also effective for alleviating facial pain and promoting overall relaxation.

P6 (Nei Guan): This point is often used in combination with other points to address issues like motion sickness and anxiety.

ST36 (Zu San Li): Known for its ability to boost energy, it's frequently used to enhance vitality and support overall health.

BL23 (Shen Shu): This point is essential for addressing lower back issues and supporting kidney function.

By focusing on these and other key points, Shiatsu practitioners can effectively address various health concerns and promote a sense of balance and well-being.

Each point has its unique benefits and can be used alone or in combination with other points to achieve comprehensive results.

CHAPTER TWO

BASIC SHIATSU TECHNIQUES

Shiatsu massage, an ancient Japanese bodywork technique, relies on the application of pressure along specific points and meridians on the body to promote balance and health.

To master Shiatsu, it's essential to understand and practice its basic techniques, which include applying pressure, stretching, and rotating joints.

Begin with the foundational technique of thumb pressure. This involves using your thumb to apply consistent pressure to specific points along the body's energy pathways or meridians.

Ensure that your thumb is properly aligned and that the pressure is firm yet comfortable for the recipient. This technique helps in stimulating energy flow and releasing muscle tension.

Another fundamental technique is palm pressure, where you use the palm of your hand to exert pressure on larger areas of the body. This method is particularly effective for relaxing large muscle groups and improving overall circulation.

Apply your weight evenly through your palm, and adjust the pressure according to the recipient's comfort level.

Palm Pressure Techniques

Palm pressure is a core element in Shiatsu that allows you to address broader areas of the body efficiently. To perform palm pressure, place your palm firmly against the area you wish to treat, ensuring it covers a broad surface.

Start with gentle pressure and gradually increase it as needed. Use the full surface of your palm to create a more significant impact, which helps in relieving tension and promoting relaxation.

Moving your palm in slow, circular motions can further enhance the effect, as it stimulates blood flow and loosens tight muscles.

Incorporate rhythmic and flowing movements to keep the pressure consistent. This helps in preventing any abrupt changes that could cause discomfort. Pay attention to the recipient's feedback and adjust the pressure to suit their needs.

Thumb And Finger Pressure Techniques

Thumb pressure in Shiatsu involves using the thumb to apply targeted pressure on specific points along the body's meridians. This technique is crucial for addressing localized areas of tension and blockages. Use the pads of your thumbs to press firmly but gently, maintaining a steady rhythm. Apply pressure in small, circular motions to enhance the effectiveness and release muscle knots.

Finger pressure complements thumb pressure by allowing more precise control over the amount of pressure applied. Use the tips of your fingers to work on smaller areas or sensitive spots.

This technique is especially useful for working on acupressure points or areas where precision is required.

Ensure that your fingers are relaxed and aligned correctly to avoid strain. The goal is to apply pressure that is both firm and comfortable, helping to stimulate energy flow and promote healing.

Stretching And Joint Rotations

Stretching and joint rotations are essential techniques in Shiatsu that help in enhancing flexibility and relieve tension.

Stretching involves gently pulling or extending specific body parts to improve the range of motion and release tight muscles. Start with slow, controlled stretches and gradually increase the intensity as needed. Focus on major muscle groups and ensure that the stretches are comfortable and do not cause pain.

Joint rotations involve moving the joints through their full range of motion. This technique helps in loosening up stiff joints and improving overall mobility. Perform rotations slowly and methodically, ensuring that each movement is smooth and controlled. This can be particularly beneficial for individuals with joint stiffness or limited mobility.

Incorporate both stretching and joint rotations into your Shiatsu practice to provide a comprehensive approach to relaxation and muscle relief.

Breathing Techniques For Relaxation

Breathing techniques play a crucial role in Shiatsu, as they help promote relaxation and enhance the effectiveness of the massage.

Encourage the recipient to engage in deep, diaphragmatic breathing. This involves inhaling deeply through the nose, allowing the abdomen to expand, and exhaling slowly through the mouth. This type of breathing helps in reducing stress, calming the nervous system, and improving the overall experience of the massage.

Incorporate breathing exercises into your Shiatsu sessions by synchronizing your movements with the recipient's breath. For instance, apply pressure during the inhalation and release it during exhalation. This coordination enhances the flow of energy and promotes a deeper sense of relaxation.

Combining Techniques For Effective Treatment

Combining different Shiatsu techniques can enhance the overall effectiveness of the treatment and address various aspects of the recipient's well-being.

Start by integrating palm and thumb pressure techniques to cover both broad and targeted areas. Begin with palm pressure to relax large muscle groups, followed by thumb pressure to address specific points of tension.

Incorporate stretching and joint rotations to complement the pressure techniques. Use stretching to improve flexibility and joint rotations to enhance mobility. This combination provides a holistic approach to relaxation and muscle relief.

Finally, integrate breathing techniques throughout the session. Encourage deep breathing to support the body's natural healing processes and enhance the overall effectiveness of the Shiatsu treatment.

By combining these techniques, you create a comprehensive Shiatsu experience that addresses multiple aspects of physical and emotional well-being.

CHAPTER THREE

SELF-SHIATSU TECHNIQUES

Shiatsu massage is a profound and effective form of bodywork originating from Japan. Self-Shiatsu allows you to harness its benefits independently, focusing on relieving tension and promoting overall wellness. The techniques involve applying pressure to specific points on your body to stimulate energy flow and release blockages.

To begin, use your fingers, palms, or thumbs to apply steady, gentle pressure on various acupressure points. These points are typically located along the energy pathways, or meridians, of the body. You can use different techniques such as pressing, kneading, or rotating movements. Each technique is aimed at enhancing the flow of energy, improving circulation, and relieving muscle tightness.

For effective results, ensure your movements are deliberate and controlled. Avoid applying excessive pressure, as this can lead to discomfort or strain. Instead, focus on gradually increasing pressure as needed and listen to your body's feedback.

Preparing For Self-Shiatsu

Proper preparation is key to a successful self-Shiatsu practice. Start by creating a calm and comfortable environment where you can relax without distractions. Find a quiet space with sufficient lighting and a comfortable surface, such as a yoga mat or a soft carpet.

Dress in loose, comfortable clothing to ensure ease of movement. It is also beneficial to practice self-Shiatsu on an empty stomach or at least a few hours after a meal. This allows for better energy flow and minimizes discomfort.

Before beginning, perform some gentle stretching or warm-up exercises to loosen up your muscles. This will help you to be more relaxed and prepared for the self-Shiatsu session. Make sure to have a water bottle nearby, as staying hydrated is essential for the body's recovery process.

Key Areas For Self-Treatment

Identifying and focusing on key areas for self-treatment can significantly enhance the effectiveness of your Shiatsu practice. Commonly targeted areas include the shoulders, neck, lower back, and legs.

For the shoulders and neck, apply pressure to points where you feel tightness or discomfort. These areas are often prone to stress and tension, and regular self-Shiatsu can provide relief. For the lower back, focus on points along the spine and around the lumbar region. This can help alleviate lower back pain and improve overall mobility.

Legs, especially the calves and thighs, are also important areas to address. Applying pressure to these areas can enhance circulation and reduce muscle fatigue. Remember to work both sides of the body equally to maintain balance and symmetry.

Step-By-Step Self-Shiatsu Routine

Developing a structured self-Shiatsu routine can help you consistently reap the benefits of this practice. Start by allocating a specific time each day or week for your Shiatsu session, aiming for 15 to 30 minutes each time.

Begin your routine with a brief warm-up to prepare your body.

Next, move on to applying pressure to the key areas identified earlier. Start with gentle pressure and gradually increase as you become more comfortable. Use both hands to apply pressure to each acupressure point, holding for about 30 seconds to a minute before moving on to the next point.

Incorporate stretching exercises between Shiatsu techniques to enhance flexibility and muscle relaxation.

Finish your routine with a few minutes of deep breathing and relaxation to help integrate the effects of the massage.

Using Tools for Self-Shiatsu

While self-Shiatsu can be performed effectively using just your hands, various tools can enhance the experience and target specific areas more precisely.

Tools such as Shiatsu balls, massage sticks, and foam rollers can be particularly useful.

Shiatsu balls are designed to help apply even pressure to acupressure points, allowing for deeper and more focused treatment.

Massage sticks and foam rollers can be used to work on larger muscle groups, such as the thighs and calves, providing a more extensive massage.

When using these tools, ensure you follow the manufacturer's instructions and use them gently to avoid overexerting yourself.

Integrate tool-based techniques into your routine as needed, focusing on areas that require extra attention.

Tips For Effective Self-Practice

To maximize the benefits of your self-Shiatsu practice, consider the following tips:

Consistency: Make self-Shiatsu a regular part of your wellness routine. Consistent practice helps maintain the balance of energy and muscle relaxation.

Listen to Your Body: Pay attention to your body's signals during the practice. Adjust the pressure and techniques based on your comfort level and needs.

Hydrate: Drink plenty of water before and after your self-Shiatsu session to support muscle recovery and overall hydration.

Create a Relaxing Environment: Ensure your practice space is calm and free from interruptions. This will help you focus and maximize the relaxation benefits.

Stay Educated: Continue learning about Shiatsu techniques and updates to improve your practice.

Books, online resources, and professional workshops can provide valuable insights and enhance your skills.

By following these tips, you can ensure that your self-Shiatsu practice is both effective and enjoyable, contributing positively to your overall health and well-being.

CHAPTER FOUR

SHIATSU FOR COMMON AILMENTS

Shiatsu massage, a traditional Japanese therapy, offers a holistic approach to treating a variety of common ailments.

By applying gentle pressure to specific points along the body's meridians, Shiatsu can help balance energy flow, alleviate pain, and promote overall well-being. Let's explore how Shiatsu can be effectively used for some common health concerns.

Shiatsu For Headaches And Migraines

Headaches and migraines can be debilitating, but Shiatsu offers relief by addressing the underlying causes and alleviating symptoms. This technique focuses on pressure points around the head, neck, and shoulders, which are often tense or blocked. For instance, applying pressure to the "Yintang" point, located between the eyebrows, can help ease frontal headaches.

Techniques like gentle kneading and stretching of the neck and shoulders can also relieve tension that may contribute to migraines. Shiatsu helps to relax the muscles, improve circulation, and balance the energy flow, reducing the frequency and severity of headaches.

Shiatsu For Back Pain

Back pain is a prevalent issue that can significantly impact daily life. Shiatsu can be highly effective in addressing both acute and chronic back pain.

The therapist will use a combination of pressure, stretching, and rhythmic tapping to release tension in the back muscles. Points along the Bladder meridian, which runs parallel to the spine, are commonly targeted. By focusing on these points, Shiatsu helps to release tight muscles, improve posture, and enhance flexibility.

Additionally, Shiatsu promotes better alignment of the spine, which can reduce strain and prevent future back pain.

Shiatsu For Digestive Issues

Digestive issues, such as bloating, constipation, or abdominal pain, can often be managed with Shiatsu. The technique involves applying pressure to points along the Stomach and Spleen meridians, which are associated with digestive health.

For instance, the "Zusanli" point, located on the lower leg, can help improve digestion and alleviate abdominal discomfort.

Gentle abdominal massage techniques, including circular motions and deep breathing exercises, can also promote better digestion and relieve symptoms of indigestion and bloating. Shiatsu helps to stimulate the digestive organs, enhance circulation, and restore balance to the digestive system.

Shiatsu For Anxiety And Stress

In today's fast-paced world, stress and anxiety are common concerns. Shiatsu massage offers a natural way to manage these issues by promoting relaxation and emotional balance. The therapist will focus on points along the Liver and Heart meridians, which are related to emotional well-being.

Techniques such as gentle stretching and pressure application help to release built-up tension and calm the nervous system.

Shiatsu encourages the production of endorphins, which are natural mood lifters and promote a sense of calm and relaxation.

Regular sessions can help to manage stress levels, improve sleep quality, and enhance overall emotional resilience.

Customizing Shiatsu For Personal Needs

Every individual has unique health needs, and Shiatsu can be tailored to address personal concerns effectively.

Customizing Shiatsu involves assessing the client's specific symptoms, health history, and preferences to create a personalized treatment plan.

This may include focusing on particular areas of tension, adjusting the pressure techniques used, or incorporating additional therapies such as aromatherapy or acupressure.

By customizing the approach, Shiatsu can address specific issues such as chronic pain, sports injuries, or post-operative recovery. `

The goal is to provide a holistic treatment that supports the individual's overall health and well-being, ensuring a more effective and satisfying experience.

CHAPTER FIVE

SHIATSU FOR MENTAL HEALTH

Shiatsu massage, a traditional Japanese therapy, is renowned for its benefits beyond physical health, particularly in enhancing mental well-being. By applying pressure to specific points on the body, Shiatsu helps to balance the body's energy, or Qi, which can significantly impact mental health. Regular Shiatsu sessions can alleviate symptoms of stress, anxiety, and depression, making it a valuable tool for maintaining mental clarity and emotional balance.

The Mind-Body Connection In Shiatsu

Shiatsu is based on the principle that mental and physical health are interconnected. The therapy focuses on the body's energy pathways, known as meridians, which are linked to various organs and emotional states. By stimulating these points, Shiatsu helps to release blocked energy and restore balance, promoting a sense of calm and emotional stability. This holistic approach acknowledges that mental well-being is influenced by physical health, and vice versa, creating a comprehensive path to overall wellness.

Techniques To Alleviate Anxiety And Depression

Shiatsu offers several techniques specifically designed to address anxiety and depression. One effective method is acupressure, where gentle yet firm pressure is applied to specific points on the body to release tension and promote relaxation. Another technique involves stretching and gentle manipulations, which help to ease muscle tension and improve circulation, contributing to a reduction in anxiety levels. By targeting the areas associated with stress and emotional imbalance, Shiatsu can help individuals feel more grounded and emotionally balanced.

Shiatsu For Improved Sleep

Sleep disturbances are often linked to stress and anxiety. Shiatsu can be particularly beneficial for improving sleep quality. Techniques such as rhythmic pressure and gentle stretching help to relax the body and mind, making it easier to fall asleep and stay asleep.

Additionally, Shiatsu can help to regulate the body's internal clock by balancing the energy flow and calming the nervous system. Regular Shiatsu sessions can create a sense of relaxation and peace, contributing to more restful and uninterrupted sleep.

Enhancing Mental Clarity And Focus

Mental clarity and focus are essential for productivity and overall cognitive function. Shiatsu can enhance these cognitive abilities by promoting relaxation and reducing mental fatigue.

Techniques such as targeted pressure on specific points help to improve blood flow and oxygenation to the brain, which can enhance cognitive function and concentration.

By reducing stress and promoting mental relaxation, Shiatsu helps individuals maintain sharp focus and clarity in their daily activities.

Building a Regular Practice for Mental Well-being

Incorporating Shiatsu into a regular wellness routine can significantly benefit mental health. To build a sustainable practice, start by scheduling regular Shiatsu sessions, whether with a professional therapist or through self-massage techniques. Establishing a routine allows for consistent energy balancing and stress reduction.

Additionally, integrating Shiatsu techniques into daily life, such as self-massage or simple stretching exercises, can reinforce the benefits and contribute to long-term mental well-being. Consistency is key to achieving and maintaining the positive effects of Shiatsu on mental health.

CHAPTER SIX

SHIATSU FOR SPORTS AND PHYSICAL ACTIVITY

Shiatsu, a traditional Japanese form of massage therapy, is particularly beneficial for athletes and individuals engaged in regular physical activity.

This therapeutic technique focuses on balancing the body's energy and promoting overall well-being through the application of pressure along specific points and meridians.

For those who lead an active lifestyle, Shiatsu can play a crucial role in enhancing performance, aiding recovery, and preventing injuries.

Benefits Of Shiatsu For Athletes

Athletes can greatly benefit from Shiatsu due to its comprehensive approach to physical and mental health.

Shiatsu helps improve circulation, which ensures that nutrients and oxygen reach the muscles more efficiently, aiding in faster recovery and enhanced performance.

The technique also targets tension and tightness in the muscles, which can help alleviate chronic pain or stiffness that might hinder athletic performance.

Moreover, Shiatsu can enhance overall flexibility by releasing tightness in the muscle tissues and improving joint mobility. The practice also aids in reducing stress and anxiety, which can contribute to better focus and mental clarity during training and competitions. Regular Shiatsu sessions can contribute to a more balanced and resilient body, enabling athletes to train harder and recover quicker.

Pre- And Post-Workout Shiatsu

Incorporating Shiatsu into your pre-and post-workout routine can be incredibly advantageous.

Pre-workout Shiatsu focuses on preparing the muscles for physical exertion. By stimulating the body's energy pathways and relaxing the muscles, Shiatsu helps to enhance circulation and flexibility, making it easier to engage in strenuous activities.

This preemptive approach reduces the likelihood of muscle strain and injury by ensuring that the body is adequately prepared for the physical demands of exercise.

Post-workout Shiatsu is equally important as it aids in muscle recovery and reduces soreness. After a workout, muscles can become tight and inflamed due to lactic acid build-up.

Shiatsu helps to alleviate this by promoting lymphatic drainage and increasing blood flow to the affected areas.

This process assists in flushing out toxins and speeding up the healing process, helping you feel rejuvenated and ready for your next session.

Techniques For Muscle Recovery

Shiatsu employs various techniques that are particularly effective for muscle recovery. One such technique is deep tissue pressure, which targets the deeper layers of muscles and connective tissues.

By applying focused pressure to specific points, Shiatsu helps to release muscle knots and alleviate chronic tension, which is crucial for effective recovery.

Another technique used in Shiatsu is stretching and joint mobilization. This involves gently stretching the muscles and moving the joints through their full range of motion.

This not only helps to increase flexibility but also reduces muscle stiffness and improves overall joint function. This technique is particularly beneficial for athletes who experience tightness or discomfort after intense physical activity.

Shiatsu also incorporates acupressure, which involves applying pressure to specific points along the body's meridians. This technique helps to stimulate the body's natural healing processes and enhance circulation, further aiding in muscle recovery and overall well-being.

Enhancing Flexibility And Performance

Flexibility is a key component of athletic performance, and Shiatsu can significantly contribute to improving it.

By targeting specific points and meridians, Shiatsu helps to release tension in the muscles and connective tissues, leading to an increased range of motion and enhanced flexibility.

This can be especially beneficial for athletes involved in sports that require a high degree of flexibility, such as gymnastics or martial arts.

In addition to improving flexibility, Shiatsu can also enhance overall performance. By addressing muscle imbalances and reducing stress, Shiatsu helps to create a more balanced and well-functioning body.

This not only improves physical performance but also supports mental focus and concentration, which are crucial for success in any athletic endeavor.

Preventing Sports Injuries With Shiatsu

Injury prevention is a critical aspect of athletic training, and Shiatsu can play a significant role in this area.

Regular Shiatsu sessions help to maintain optimal muscle and joint function by addressing areas of tightness and imbalance. By promoting proper alignment and reducing muscle tension, Shiatsu helps to minimize the risk of common sports injuries, such as strains and sprains.

Additionally, Shiatsu aids in improving overall body awareness and proprioception, which can help athletes recognize and address potential issues before they lead to injuries.

By incorporating Shiatsu into a regular training regimen, athletes can enhance their body's resilience and reduce the likelihood of injury, ensuring a safer and more effective training experience.

CHAPTER SEVEN

PARTNER SHIATSU TECHNIQUES

Partner Shiatsu is an enriching practice where two individuals work together to achieve mutual relaxation and well-being.

To get started, it's essential to understand the basic techniques involved. Begin with the thumb and palm pressure, where one partner uses their thumbs to apply gentle but firm pressure to specific points on the other partner's body. This technique helps release tension and promote energy flow.

Another crucial technique is the knuckle press, which involves using the knuckles to apply pressure in circular motions.

This method is effective for targeting deeper muscle layers and alleviating stiffness. Don't forget the elbow press, where you use the elbows to deliver more concentrated pressure on tense areas. This technique is especially useful for areas like the back and shoulders.

Incorporating stretching techniques can also enhance the Shiatsu experience. One partner can gently stretch the other's arms or legs to improve flexibility and relaxation.

Ensure that all techniques are performed with a focus on the partner's comfort and consent, adjusting pressure and intensity as needed.

Preparing For Partner Shiatsu

Proper preparation is key to a successful Partner Shiatsu session. Begin by setting up a comfortable space where both partners can relax. Use a soft mat or blanket to provide cushioning and ensure the area is free from distractions.

Dress comfortably in loose clothing that allows for easy movement and pressure application.

Before starting, it's crucial to communicate with your partner about any specific areas of discomfort or tension.

This helps tailor the session to their needs. Perform a brief warm-up to prepare the muscles and joints for the massage.

Gentle stretching or light movements can help ease stiffness and enhance the effectiveness of the Shiatsu techniques.

Additionally, ensure both partners are hydrated and have had a light meal before the session. This helps avoid any discomfort that might arise from a full stomach or dehydration.

Basic Partner Shiatsu Routines

When performing Basic Partner Shiatsu routines, start with a simple warm-up routine. This could include gentle stretching or light pressure along the back and shoulders. Follow this with a sequence of pressure points—applying steady pressure to key points on the body, such as the shoulders, neck, and back.

Incorporate long strokes to promote relaxation and improve blood circulation. Using the palms, glide smoothly over the back, applying even pressure.

Transition into circular motions with your fingers or palms to work on specific tension spots.

Finish the routine with a relaxation phase, where both partners lie down and focus on deep breathing. This helps to integrate the benefits of the massage and allows the body to fully relax.

Communicating With Your Partner

Effective communication is vital in Partner Shiatsu to ensure a positive and comfortable experience for both individuals. Discuss preferences and any areas of discomfort before starting the session.

This can include preferred pressure levels, specific areas needing attention, or any physical limitations.

During the session, maintain an open line of communication by checking in regularly with your partner.

Ask how the pressure feels and if any adjustments are needed. Encourage them to express their needs and comfort level at all times.

After the session, provide feedback to each other about what worked well and any areas that might need improvement. This helps in refining the techniques and ensuring that both partners benefit from the Shiatsu practice.

Creating A Relaxing Environment

Creating a relaxing environment enhances the effectiveness of Partner Shiatsu and contributes to a soothing experience. Start by choosing a quiet, peaceful space free from external noise and interruptions. Soft, ambient music can help create a calming atmosphere.

Consider using essential oils or aromatherapy to add a sensory dimension to the session. Scents like lavender or eucalyptus can promote relaxation and improve the overall experience.

Additionally, adjust the lighting to be soft and gentle, avoiding harsh or bright lights.

Ensure the space is warm and comfortable. Use blankets or cushions to provide additional comfort and support during the session. A relaxing environment helps both partners unwind and fully enjoy the benefits of the Shiatsu practice.

Benefits Of Partner Shiatsu

Partner Shiatsu offers numerous benefits, both physical and emotional. Physically, it helps in relieving muscle tension and reducing stress. The application of pressure to key points stimulates blood circulation and promotes the flow of energy throughout the body.

Emotionally, Partner Shiatsu fosters a sense of connection and well-being. The act of giving and receiving massage strengthens the bond between partners and provides a shared experience of relaxation. It can also enhance communication and empathy, as both partners become more attuned to each other's needs and responses.

Additionally, engaging in Partner Shiatsu can contribute to improved flexibility and posture, as the techniques often involve stretching and gentle manipulation of the body.

 Regular practice can lead to a more balanced and relaxed state, benefiting both partners in their daily lives.

CHAPTER EIGHT

COMMON CONCERNS AND FAQS

Will Shiatsu Massage Hurt?

One of the most common concerns about Shiatsu massage is whether it will be painful. Shiatsu involves applying pressure to specific points on the body, which can sometimes cause discomfort, especially if there are tight muscles or blocked energy pathways.

However, a skilled practitioner will adjust the pressure to your comfort level, ensuring that the experience is therapeutic rather than painful.

It's important to communicate openly with your therapist about any discomfort you feel during the session.

Is Shiatsu Suitable for Everyone?

Shiatsu is generally safe for most people, but there are some exceptions. Individuals with certain medical conditions, such as severe osteoporosis, open wounds, or recent surgery, should avoid Shiatsu. Pregnant women should also consult with their healthcare provider before undergoing Shiatsu therapy, as certain pressure points may be contraindicated during pregnancy. Always disclose your medical history to your practitioner to ensure that Shiatsu is safe for you.

How Should I Prepare for a Shiatsu Session?

Preparing for a Shiatsu session is straightforward. Wear loose, comfortable clothing that allows for easy movement. Avoid eating a heavy meal or drinking alcohol before your appointment. It's also a good idea to arrive a few minutes early to relax and fill out any necessary paperwork. Keeping hydrated before and after your session can enhance the benefits of the massage.

Addressing Common Misconceptions

Shiatsu Is Just a Fancy Name for Massage

Shiatsu is often mistaken for just another type of massage, but it is much more than that. Shiatsu is rooted in traditional Japanese medicine and aims to balance the body's energy flow, or "Qi," through pressure points, stretches, and joint rotations. Unlike conventional massages that primarily focus on muscle relaxation, Shiatsu works on a deeper level to harmonize the body's energy system, promoting overall health and well-being.

You Need to Undress for Shiatsu

A common misconception is that you need to undress for a Shiatsu session. Shiatsu is typically performed with the client fully clothed. The practitioner uses their hands, thumbs, elbows, and knees to apply pressure through your clothing. This approach not only respects personal boundaries but also allows for seamless transitions between different techniques and positions during the session.

How Often Should You Get Shiatsu?

Determining the Right Frequency

The ideal frequency of Shiatsu sessions depends on your individual needs and health goals. For general wellness and stress relief, a session every two to four weeks may suffice. However, if you're dealing with chronic pain, high-stress levels, or specific health issues, more frequent sessions, such as once a week, might be beneficial. Your practitioner can help you determine a schedule that best supports your health objectives.

Listening to Your Body

It's important to listen to your body and adjust the frequency of your sessions based on how you feel. After a Shiatsu session, take note of any changes in your energy levels, pain, or overall well-being. If you notice significant improvements, you might be able to extend the time between sessions. Conversely, if your symptoms persist or worsen, you may need more frequent treatments.

What To Expect During A Session

Initial Consultation

Your first Shiatsu session will typically begin with a brief consultation. The practitioner will ask about your medical history, current health concerns, and specific areas of discomfort. This information helps tailor the session to your needs and ensures a safe and effective treatment.

The Treatment Process

During the session, you will lie on a futon mat on the floor, or sometimes on a massage table. The practitioner will apply pressure to various points on your body using their hands, thumbs, elbows, and knees. The pressure can be gentle or firm, depending on your comfort level and therapeutic needs. Stretching and joint rotation may also be incorporated to enhance the effects of the treatment.

Post-Session Feelings

After a Shiatsu session, it's normal to feel a range of sensations. Some people feel deeply relaxed and rejuvenated, while others may experience mild soreness or fatigue as their body adjusts. Drinking plenty of water and resting can help alleviate any temporary discomfort. Over time, regular Shiatsu sessions can lead to long-lasting improvements in your physical and mental well-being.

Contraindications And Safety Measures

When to Avoid Shiatsu

There are certain conditions where Shiatsu may not be appropriate. If you have severe osteoporosis, open wounds, or recent surgery, it's best to avoid Shiatsu. People with certain cardiovascular conditions or infectious diseases should also consult their healthcare provider before receiving Shiatsu. Pregnant women should inform their practitioner, as some pressure points may need to be avoided or modified.

Safety Precautions

To ensure a safe and effective Shiatsu experience, always inform your practitioner of your medical history and any current health concerns. This includes any medications you are taking, as certain conditions and treatments may require modifications to the Shiatsu techniques used. A qualified practitioner will adjust the session to accommodate your needs and ensure your safety.

Finding A Qualified Practitioner

Credentials and Training

When looking for a Shiatsu practitioner, it's important to verify their credentials and training. Look for practitioners who have completed a recognized Shiatsu training program and are certified by a reputable organization. Certification ensures that they have received comprehensive training in anatomy, physiology, and Shiatsu techniques.

Personal Recommendations

Personal recommendations can be a valuable resource when searching for a qualified Shiatsu practitioner. Ask friends, family, or healthcare providers if they can recommend someone they trust. Online reviews and testimonials can also provide insights into the practitioner's skills and professionalism.

Initial Consultation

Before committing to regular sessions, consider scheduling an initial consultation with the practitioner. This allows you to discuss your health concerns, ask questions, and get a feel for their approach and demeanor. A good practitioner will listen attentively, provide clear explanations, and make you feel comfortable and confident in your care.